(Intentionally left blank

Finding Wellness in a Pandemic and Beyond

Sherri James, MD
Published by: BMI Wellness Concepts, PLLC

INTRODUCTION

What is Wellness?

Health is a state of mind and body. Wellness is an integrated state of being and making intentional choices toward a healthy and fulfilling life. The Wellness Quotient is an indicator of an individual's well-being based on eight tenets of wellness: Intellectual, Social, Spiritual, Emotional, Physical, Environmental, Occupational, and Financial.

Your Wellness Quotient (WQ) is a fluid number that changes depending on current circumstances. It can change according to what's going on in the world we live in, especially in a pandemic and political upheaval.

The COVID-19 global pandemic and the Black Lives Matter (BLM) Movement have presented the world with many different challenges.

While we are all concerned with staying safe and healthy during this difficult time, it is not a time to forget about your overall wellness. The World Health Organization says wellness is more than being free from illness. It is a dynamic process of change and growth and a state of complete physical, mental, and social well-being, and not merely the absence of disease or infirmity.

This book is a compilation of blogs created during the first outbreak of the COVID-19 pandemic. Use it to determine your WQ. *Finding Wellness in a Pandemic and Beyond,* Sherri James, MD, and BMI Wellness Concepts hope to empower people to **Get Well Be Well Stay Well**.

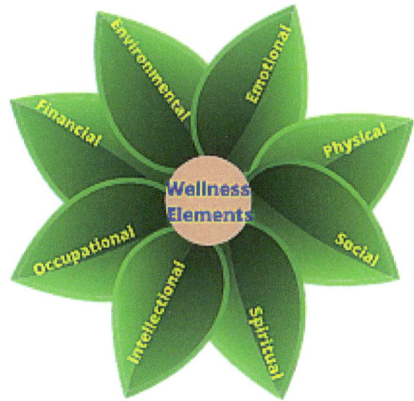

INTELLECTUAL WELLNESS

Table Of Contents

INTELLECTUAL WELLNESS

On the Road to Wellness Be Sure to Find Ways to Achieve Intellectual Wellness

As we travel along the the wellness journey, one important element is the state of our mind, our intellect, and our abilities to create, reason, and learn new things. Our intellectual wellness is critical in our overall wellness.

What is Intellectual Wellness?

Intellectual wellness is the opening of our mind to new experiences and new ideas, expanding our knowledge, refining our skills, and participating in various activities that stimulate thought, enhance cultural understanding, embrace artistic expression, foster creativity, spark curiosity, develop mindfulness, and encourage lifelong learning.

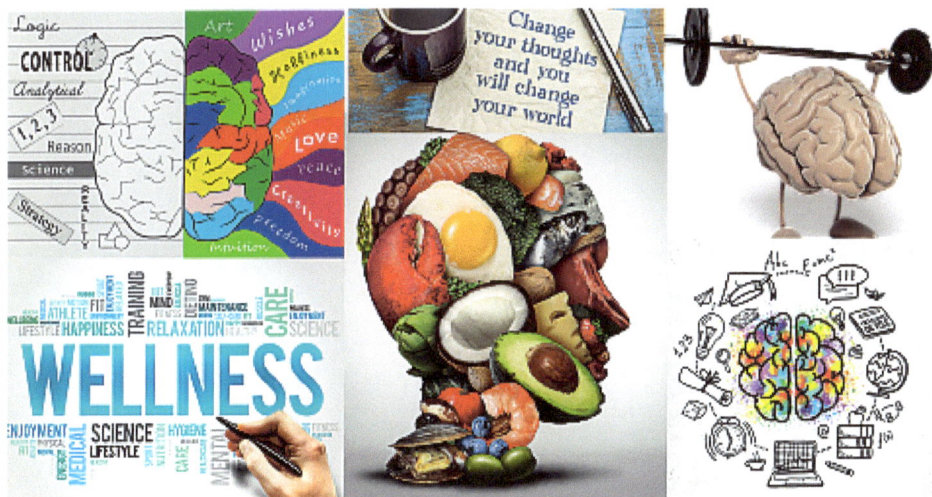

INTELLECTUAL WELLNESS

- **Why is Intellectual Wellness Important? It...**
  - Encourages learning.
  - Inspires exploration.
  - Stimulates curiosity.
  - Enhances motivation.
  - Feeds open-mindedness.
  - Launches critical thinking.
  - Builds new skills.
  - Fuels creativity.
  - Develops problem-solving.
  - Increases knowledge.
  - Facilitates understanding.
  - Fosters appreciation of differences.
  - Sparks artistic expression.
  - Forges dialog and communication pathways.
  - Extends friendships
  - Creates connections
  - Bridges networks.

INTELLECTUAL WELLNESS

- **How to Improve Intellectual Wellness?**
  - Be Open-Minded.
  - Participate in Active Listening.
  - Travel to new destinations.
  - Learn about different cultures, races, and ethnicities.
  - Read books, articles, news, and blogs.
  - Listen to podcasts.
  - Engage in community activities.
  - Talk to people with different backgrounds and experiences.
  - Try a new hobby.
  - Engage in artistic endeavors.
  - Take a class or learn a new skill.
  - Teach a class.
  - Be a mentor.
  - Share your knowledge or expertise,
  - Discover your playfulness.
  - Meet new people.
  - Volunteer.
  - Keep a journal.
  - Read for fun.
  - Do crossword and other puzzles.
  - Learn a new language.
  - Research a topic or brush-up on history.
  - Write an article, a blog, a short story, a poem, a novel, or screenplay.

IWQ

INTELLECTUAL WELLNESS QUOTIENT (IWQ)

INSTRUCTIONS: Answer each question accurately. Each answer that describes you best, will be scored on a scale of 1 to 4: 1 = Nope, that is not me. 2 = Sometimes, that describes me. 3 = Often that is me. 4 = Yes, that's definitely me!

INTELLECTUAL - Intellectual Wellness has to do with how curious you are and how open you are to learn or experience new things. It includes embracing or tackling new challenges and finding ways to develop additional skills. It also has to do with your ability to share your knowledge and expertise with others.

1. I am curious about new topics, different cultures, and visiting places outside my community, region, or country.
__1___ No, that's not me, I am comfortable with what I know and where I live.
__2___ Sometimes, I am open to learning new things, meeting new people, and seeing new places.
__3___ Often I seek to learn about people, places, and cultures that are different from my life.
__4___ Yes! I want to experience as much as I can from many different people, cultures, and sources.

2. I regularly seek out activities that challenge my brain, stimulate my curiosity, or offer inspiration.
__1___ No, that's not me. I'm not one to really seek new experiences.
__2___ Sometimes I look for ways to make me think about things or see things from a different perspective.
__3___ Often I am curious, and I look for new ways of thinking about situations.
__4___ Yes, I constantly seek new challenges and my brain thrives on curiosity and inspiration!

3. I enjoy sharing my knowledge and expertise with others as a way of helping people.
__1___ No, that's not me. I don't feel like I have any knowledge or expertise that is valuable to others.
__2___ Sometimes, I like to share what I know or what I have experienced with others.
__3___ Often I look for ways that I can help people with my knowledge, expertise, and experiences.
__4___ Yes, I find satisfaction that my knowledge and expertise can help others.

4. When I learn new information, I am open to changing my mind or seeing a different perspective.
__1___ No, that's not me. I am comfortable knowing that I know what I need to know.
__2___ Sometimes, I am open to learning new information and considering a new way of thinking.
__3___ Often I seek out new ways of thinking about situations.
__4___ Yes! I want to learn new information, hear different perspectives, and challenge my beliefs for my own growth.

5. When I make a mistake, I own it and I use it as a way to learn from it.
__1___ No, that's not me – I am sure that something or someone caused me to flub up.
__2___ Sometimes, I accept the errors I make and I'm willing to try to find a lesson in that mistake.
__3___ Often I accept my failings, and I make changes to prevent similar mistakes in the future.
__4___ Yes, I know when I mess up and I want to make sure that I don't do it again.

TOTAL FOR THIS SECTION ____

SOCIAL WELLNESS

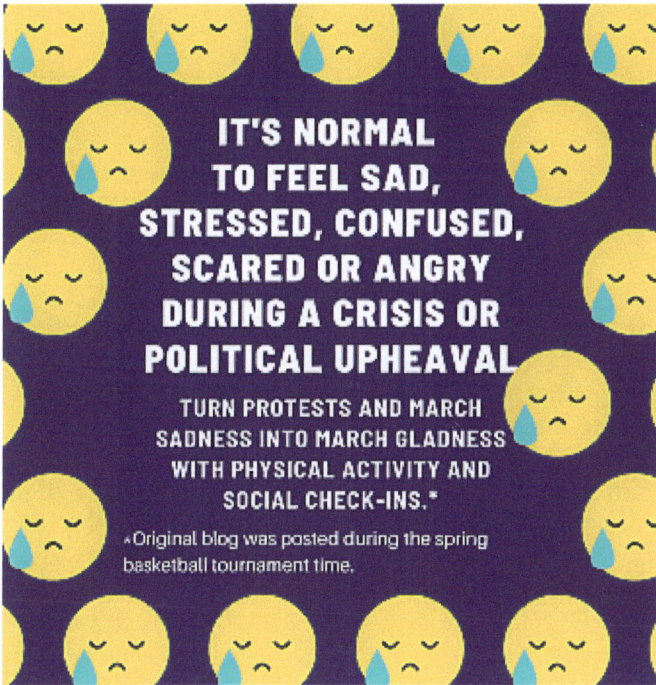

IT'S NORMAL TO FEEL SAD, STRESSED, CONFUSED, SCARED OR ANGRY DURING A CRISIS OR POLITICAL UPHEAVAL

TURN PROTESTS AND MARCH SADNESS INTO MARCH GLADNESS WITH PHYSICAL ACTIVITY AND SOCIAL CHECK-INS.*

*Original blog was posted during the spring basketball tournament time.

What is Social Wellness?

Social wellness refers to the relationships we cultivate and the way we interact and connect with others.

Often we socialize in gyms, over meals in restaurants, at backyard BBQs, Happy Hours, protests like Black Lives Matter movement, cultural events like Cinco De Mayo, Juneteenth, July 4th celebrations, and other gatherings.

In this new era of uncertainty and mandatory social distancing in an effort to prevent the spread of the Coronavirus or COVID-19, most of us are at a loss of how to cope with the disruption in our daily lives. By prohibiting direct face-to-face interactions, closing schools, and suspending sports, social gatherings, meetups, parties, dinners out with friends, weddings, worship services, group workouts, gym classes, and through protests while wearing masks, it is understandable if you are feeling a lot of sadness and anxiety right now.

SOCIAL WELLNESS

Since most gyms are closed to large gatherings and you can't enjoy your favorite spin class or Zumba workout, why not participate in a group exercise on Zoom? Here are some ways to keep you physically well when you can't get to the gym and to stay socially close while maintaining physical distances.

- **Lunges** - Side, Front/Back and Curtsy Lunges - step to the left, bring the right leg at an angle behind and bend the left knee keeping your torso upright and your arms out to the side, as if you're holding a big dress. Then do alternating intervals.
- **Squats** - for more of a workout, add in a reach up with both hands reaching for the ceiling or a jump up.
- **Mountain Climbers** - Traditionally with both hands and knees on the floor and then alternating walking one foot toward your hands and straightening the other leg/foot behind you in continuous repetitions. Modifications - can be done from standing position reaching toward the ceiling/sky and bring in the opposite knee toward your chest and alternate sides.
- **Leg Lifts** - Either from a standing, sitting, or prone position on your stomach or back.
- **Crunches** - Prone, sitting or standing - do intervals of tightening and releasing your abs. For more of a workout bend elbows toward opposite knees.
- **Calf Raises** - Standing or Sitting. Jump rope - even an imaginary one can give you a good workout!
- **Wall Sit** - Place your back against the wall and slide down into a sitting position and then hold for 60 seconds or longer - you'll feel the burn in your thighs!
- **High Knees** - Standing, or even sitting - bring your knees up toward your chest.
- **Arm Curls** - with or without hand weights or household items.
- **Run in Place** - 30 - to - 60 second intervals.
- **Shoulder Presses** - Pretend you have an orange between your shoulder blades and you need to squeeze it to get the juice out.
- **Supermans/Superwomans** - stretch out onto your stomach and stretch arms above your head and then simultaneously lift your arms and legs off the floor with your torso still. Slow neck rotations - up, down, left, right, back.

SOCIAL WELLNESS

- **Shadow Boxing** - do various number combinations for 30-second intervals with or without hand weights or household objects. Dominant hands/arms are usually stronger, so you might have to work your less dominant hand/arm a little more!

  - Boxing punch 1 (for right handers) = Left hand curled into a fist with the back of hand facing the ceiling, punch forward, like you're socking someone in the nose. (For left-handers start with your right.)
  - Boxing punch 2 (for right-handers) = Right hand curled into a fist with the back of your hand facing the ceiling, punch forward. (For left-handers this punch is with your left hand.)
  - Boxing punch 3 (for right-handers) = Left hand curled into a fist, like you are holding a mug, so the back of your hand faces left , and hook your punch as if you're hitting someone on their side (For left-handers this punch is with your right hand.)
  - Boxing punch 4 (for right handers) = Right hand curled into a fist, like you are holding a mug, so the back of your hand faces right, and hook your punch, as if you're hitting someone on their side. (Left-handers this punch is with your left hand.)
  - Boxing punch 5 (for right-handers) = Left hand curled into a fist, with the wrist facing the ceiling, punch upward. (Left-handers this punch is with your right hand.)
  - Boxing punch 6 (for right-handers) = Right hand curled into a fist, with wrist facing the ceiling, punch upward. (Left-handers this punch is with your left hand.)

Low-Calorie Snacks

Let's face it, being at home often means more time spent watching TV and snacking. So why not take advantage of your favorite TV cooking show and prepare your own snacks? Here are are some healthy snack ideas.

- **Veggies and Hummus** - carrots, broccoli, radishes, celery, peppers and hummus are filling and satisfying. (One medium carrot and 2 Tablespoons of Hummus are about 100 calories.)
- **Apples and Peanut Butter** - a small apple and about 2 Tablespoons of natural peanut butter can provide protein and nutrients. Natural peanut butter only has peanuts and salt. (This snack has about 267 calories.)
- **Coconut Chips** - Healthier than potato chips - purchased or make your own. If you do it yourself, toss unsweetened coconut flakes in melted coconut oil and bake in a 300-degree oven for 7-9 minutes. Add salt and vinegar or cinnamon and honey for a different flavor. (1/2 Cup = 315 Calories)

SOCIAL WELLNESS

- **Hard boiled egg** - provides protein, vitamin B12, vitamin A, selenium, phosphorus, and healthy fats at only 78 calories!
- **Greek Yogurt and Berries** - this snack provides protein, calcium, magnesium, and potassium, fiber, and antioxidants. Seven ounces of Greek Yogurt and 1/2 cup of blueberries = 180 calories.
- **Bananas and Nut Butter** - A sweet and salty snack that provides protein and fiber. One small banana and 2 Tablespoons of Almond Butter = 280 Calories.
- **Roasted Almonds and Dried Cherries** - a great healthy snack because almonds provide protein, fiber and magnesium and cherries are filled with fiber and Vitamin A. Recent studies show this combo can reduce the risk for heart disease and diabetes! 1/4 Cup of Almonds + 1/4 Cup of Cherries= 290 Calories.
- **Smoothies** - Tasty, flavorful, and healthy smoothies offer many options with fruits, veggies, especially greens, nuts, and Greek Yogurt, and milk and/or nut/grain beverages for protein- and nutrient-rich snacks. Calories depend upon ingredients used.
- **Homemade Trail Mix** - Choose your favorite seeds, nuts, dried fruits, dark chocolate, grains, and spices. Figure on 1/4 Cup = 140 Calories.
- **Shrimp Cocktail** - It's not just a luxurious appetizer, shrimp is packed with protein, iron, selenium, and vitamin B12. Pair it with low-calorie cocktail sauce made with horseradish, unsweetened ketchup, lemon juice, Worcestershire sauce, and hot sauce and you have a snack with a punch for only about 80 calories.
- **Tomato Stuffed with Tuna** - Tomatoes have lycopene, an antioxidant that is good for our hearts and has been shown to help prevent cancers, especially prostate cancers. One small tomato stuffed with tuna salad made with mayonnaise = 150 calories.
- **Dark Chocolate and Almond Butter** - Allow yourself a little indulgence! High quality dark chocolate is loaded with antioxidants and the protein in almond butter gives you a wonderful treat. One square of dark chocolate and one Tablespoon of almond butter = 165 calories!

Check in With Friends and Family!
Even though we are being encouraged to maintain social distances, this doesn't mean we have to stop talking to, texting, and video chatting with our friends, family, neighbors, and co-workers! We are social creatures and we need our peeps in our lives. These social engagements boost morale, improve moods, ground us, and help keep us emotionally connected.

SoWQ

SOCIAL WELLNESS QUOTIENT (SoWQ)

-Social Wellness means that you cultivated and maintain connections and relationships with family , friends, and colleagues that you are able to work through any conflicts that may arise.

1. I choose to spend time with people who know me best and with whom I am my best self.

__1___ No, that's not me, I always manage to find people in my life who don't respect me or hurt me.

__2___ Sometimes, I seek out healthy relationships with family, friends, and co-workers.

__3___ Often my family, friends, and co-workers build me up.

__4___ Yes, my family, friends, and co-workers and I are a great team.

2. I am comfortable with and appreciate my relationships within my community.

__1___ No, that's not me. My relationships are strained.

__2___ Sometimes, I feel comfortable with my relationships with family, friends, or co-workers.

__3___ Often, I seek comfort from my friends, family, and/or co-workers.

__4___ Yes, I need my friends and family and I love being a part of my community.

3. I'm comfortable in my skin and confident in my decisions.

__1___ No, that's not me – I'm a people-pleaser. I worry about what others think of me.

__2___ Sometimes, I am ruled by the need to please others.

__3___ Often, I can separate my need to always please others.

__4___ Yes, I'm a renegade. I know that I can't please everyone, and I am OK with that.

4. I am comfortable being alone.

__1___ No, that's not me. I can't stand being alone – I am very much a people person.

__2___ Sometimes, I isolate myself from friends, family, and co-workers.

__3___ Often I seek regular meetings and get-togethers with family and friends.

_4___ Yes, I may be alone, but I am not lonely.

5. I work hard to not lash out and blame others for my frustrations and anger.

__1___ No, I often blame others when I am frustrated or angry.

__2___ Sometimes, when I get frustrated or angry, I lash out at others.

__3___ Often I am able to keep frustrations and anger in check.

__4___ Yes, I take responsibility for my own actions, and I do not blame others for my frustrations and anger.

TOTAL FOR THIS SECTION ___

SPIRITUAL WELLNESS

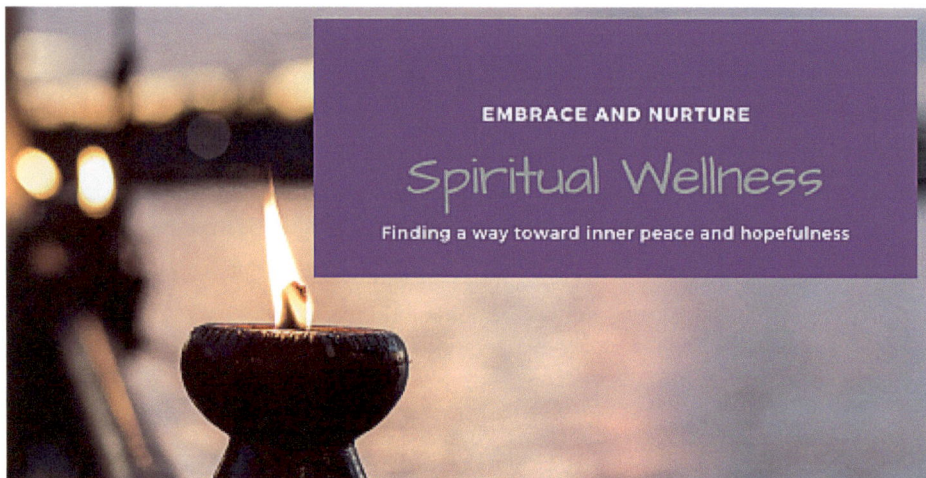

EMBRACE AND NURTURE

Spiritual Wellness

Finding a way toward inner peace and hopefulness

During the COVID-19 pandemic, our worlds have been rocked in ways that we never imagined. Many of us may feel off-kilter due to social distancing, fear, and anxiety of what the future holds for us. Part of living a life of wellness for today and every day is embracing and nurturing your spiritual wellness.

What is Spiritual Wellness?

Spiritual wellness means that you are connected to something greater than yourself. Spiritual wellness also means that you have a set of values, principles, morals and beliefs that give you a sense of purpose and meaning and they help guide your life

Benefits of Spiritual Wellness
- Improves mood and feelings of joy and happiness.
- Reduces stress levels and depression.
- Increases blood supply and metabolic activities in the body.
- Lowers blood pressure.
- Reduces blood sugar levels.
- Improves digestion and the immune system.
- Improves brain wave function, memory, and cognition.
- Provides a feeling of calmness and relaxation.

SPIRITUAL WELLNESS

Ways to Achieve Spiritual Wellness

1. **Find what gives your life meaning and purpose. Ask yourself these questions:**
   - What gives me hope?
   - How do I get through tough times?
   - Am I tolerant of other people's views? If not, how can I become more tolerant?
   - Do I expand my awareness, knowledge of, and my respect for different ethnic, racial, and religious groups?
   - Do I make time to relax and decompress?
   - Do my values guide my decisions and actions?

2. **Explore your faith and what you believe**
   - If you have never thought about a particular religion, take time to learn about the different ones.
   - Pray.

3. **Practice mindfulness for rational thinking, deeper concentration, balance, and inner peace.**
   - Meditate.
   - Be conscious and aware of your thoughts.
   - Visualize positive outcomes.
   - Refresh and revitalize your mind and body.
   - Be present and uplift yourself.

   Travel and Explore New Places.
4.
   - Take time to meet new people.
   - Learn about new cultures and ways of life.
   - Broaden your horizons.
   - Appreciate Differences.
   - Read articles, books, and watch uplifting programs.
   - Look for new or different points of view for greater empathy, understanding, and knowledge of other world views.

SPIRITUAL WELLNESS

5. Be a Mentor.
- Volunteer your time and help others.
- Share your knowledge and experiences.
- Lend a hand.
- Open your heart.
- Give respect.
- Love.
- Accept forgiveness.
- Forgive others.
- Find the good in others.
- Build people up instead of finding fault and tearing them down.
- Show gratitude and thankfulness.
- Stand for justice.
- Seek and show fair and equitable treatment to everyone.
- Advocate for the rights of others.
- Practice unity not division.
- Choose inclusion over exclusion.
- Express joy.

SpWQ

SPIRITUAL WELLNESS - SpWQ

– Spiritual wellness has to do with how meaningful your life is and whether you live a life that has purpose and is bolstered by your beliefs, faith, and morals.

1. I make choices in my life that are rewarding and fulfilling to me.
__1___ No, that's not me. I need to make better choices in my life.
__2___ Sometimes, I do things that give me a sense of accomplishment, but I could do more.
__3___ Often, I seek out ways to feel like I am making a difference in someone else's life.
__4___ Yes! I thrive on doing things that feed my soul and make me feel fulfilled.

2. I like being a part of something bigger than myself.
__1___ No, I prefer to be by myself and focus only on my own personal issues.
__2___ Sometimes, I seek out ways to be part of the larger community.
__3___ Often, I look for ways to get involved with new groups or things that are important to the community as a whole.
__4___ Yes, I thrive on being a part of meaningful activities that have a positive purpose.

3. I know what issues matters to me, and I keep them at the center of my life.
__1___ No, I struggle with finding a purpose or meaning to my life.
__2___ Sometimes I think I know what is important to me and I manage to stay on track with it. __3___ Often I am centered and focused on what's important in my life.
__4___ Yes, I have discovered my passion and I never waiver in my pursuit.

4. I wake up with a sense of purpose and direction every day.
__1___ No, that's not me at all! My life has no meaning or purpose.
__2___ Sometimes I know what I am supposed to be doing and mostly I stay on track for that goal. __3___ Often I am guided by what my purpose is in life.
__4___ Yes! I am on track and motivated to accomplish what I set out to do.

5. Everything I do coincides with my values, beliefs, faith, and life tenets.
__1___ No, that's not me – I really don't know what I value or what I believe.
__2___ Sometimes, I struggle to do things that fit within my beliefs or faith.
__3___ Often I set out to do things that align with what I value or hold dear to me.
__4___ Yes, I know what I believe and my faith in those beliefs guide and shape my life daily.

TOTAL FOR THIS SECTION ____

EMOTIONAL WELLNESS

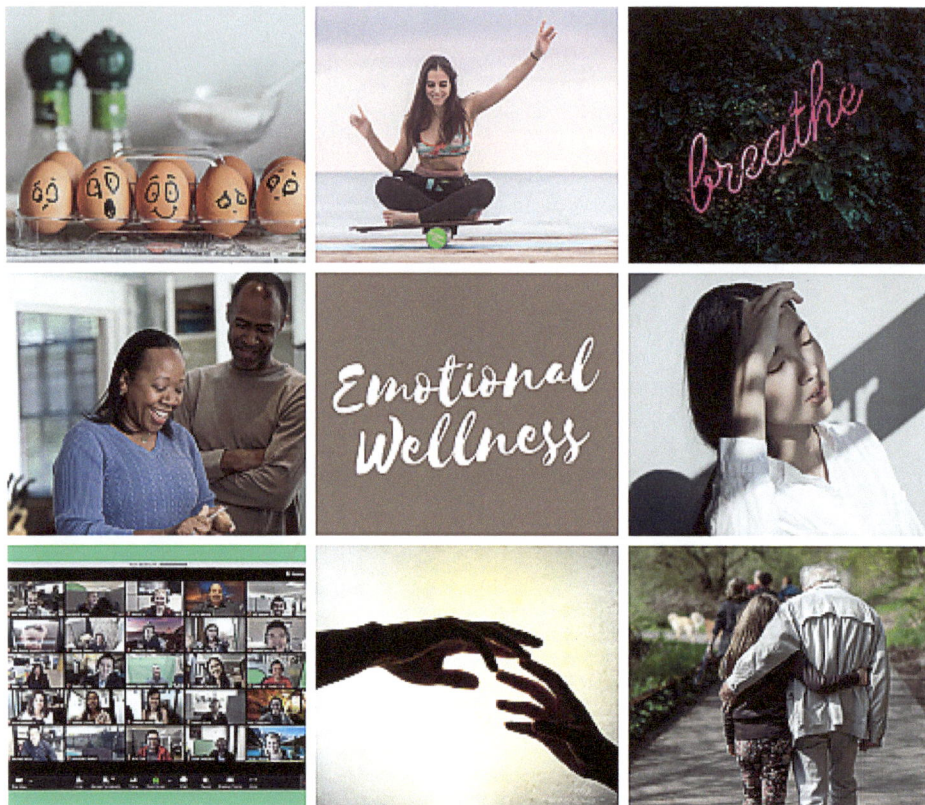

What is Emotional Wellness?

Substance Abuse and Mental Health Services Administration (SAMHSA), an agency within the U.S. Department of Health and Human Service, defines emotional wellness as the ability to cope effectively with life and to build satisfying relationships with others. People with healthy emotional wellness feel confident, in control of their feelings and behaviors, and are able to handle life challenges.

EMOTIONAL WELLNESS

Clinging to and Creating Emotional Wellness During Uncertain Times

Take a deep breath. Close your eyes and slowly exhale. Breathe in again. Let this big cleansing breath move through your body. Try it four or five more times. Doesn't that feel good? It sounds simple, but right now, we need to focus on breathing because it seems like we're all holding our collective breaths for what's next. Since the global Coronavirus Pandemic has consumed our every waking moment, most of us feel like a big ball of knots of angst, fear, sadness, confusion, anger, loneliness, isolation, and uncertainty.

The sudden and extreme changes, business shutdowns, job losses, ever-growing and seemingly unending stay-at-home orders, news updates of mounting cases of illness, and the staggering death rates have rocked our world. The missed community and family events including religious and spiritual gatherings, sports, graduations, weddings, and even funerals combined with the prospects of losing a job, health insurance, and perhaps a home can be overwhelming. It's understandable if you feel like your mind is saturated with negative thoughts, ideas and emotions.

Manage Your Stress

Stress and negativity are extremely draining. They deplete our bodies, our hearts, and our soul of energy and can rob us of our overall health and well-being.

If stress is chronic and long-term, then it can lead to mental health issues, like depression, anxiety, and personality disorders. It can also lead to many different physical issues like cardiovascular disease, heart disease, high blood pressure, abnormal heart rhythms, heart attacks, and stroke.

Just as you need to replenish your body with fluids after a workout, you also need to replenish your mind with some positive thoughts, emotions, and stay physically active.

EMOTIONAL WELLNESS

- **Take time to clear your mind.**
  - Empty your mind of negative thoughts.

- **Practice daily meditation moments - even 5-10 minutes each day!**
  - Your household may be a bit chaotic as you, your spouse, life partner, roommates, your kids, and your pets all occupy the same place 24/7. Work, school lessons, and daily living may make you feel stressed, worried, jumpy, depressed, and sad.
  - Give yourself permission to go off by yourself for a few minutes of distraction-free quiet and calm.
  - Step outside, take a short walk, or take a long shower, or a soothing bath.
  - Visualize something that makes you relax.

  - Focus on your breathing. With each breath, push out the stress, the negativity, anxiety, loneliness, sadness, and anger.
  - Breathe in positive thoughts, joyful moments, and savor beautiful, fun memories. We're all in this strange and scary situation together. We will get through these difficult times.

- **Practice Gratitude Daily.**
  - The more gratitude you pour into your life the more joyfulness you create for you and your family. Be thankful of everything large and small.

  - If you have trouble thinking of gratitude, grab a piece of paper and pen and write down 5-10 things you are thankful for in your life each day.

  - Put those scraps of paper into a jar and then pull them out at the end of the week and reflect on what you wrote down earlier in the week. You will be amazed at how much gratitude will improve your emotional well-being!

EMOTIONAL WELLNESS

- **Keep Your Physical Distance But Stay Socially Close!**
  - We are told to practice social distancing, but in reality in order to keep people healthy in the time of a global health crisis, it is prudent to keep ourselves physically distant from others, but gather in closely for our social interactions.

  - Make use of the internet, phone calls, video chats, texts, and other forms of reach-outs and check-ins on your family, friends, co-workers, faith communities, and neighbors.

  - Express love, laughter, silliness, gratitude, and appreciation of everyone in your life. These connections are what fuel our lives and sustain us through tough times.

- **Eat Healthy!**
  - If you've found yourself on an eating frenzy lately, you need to be mindful that stress can trigger the need to binge or do round-the-clock eating.

  - Look for the healthier snacks - opt for more fruits, veggies, healthy smoothies, and other nutritious items rather than feeding that emptiness you feel from the COVID-19 overload with the not-so nutritious things that start with C - cookies, candies, cakes, and chips!

- **Get Regular Exercise - at least 30 minutes a day.**
  - Get the family together for a dance party! Of course, you'll need to record it so that you can entertain the family members who aren't there or include everyone in a virtual dance party via Zoom, Skype, Google Hangouts or whatever video chat service you prefer!

  - These are great also for your regular exercise classes that you've given up on now that the gym is closed. No Excuses - Keep Moving!

  - Take a walk, or run, or ride a bike.

EMOTIONAL WELLNESS

- **Get plenty of rest.**
  - Try to stick to a regular sleep routine, even though your regular routine has changed.
  - Turn off the news. While it's important to stay informed during this pandemic, it's also good to give yourself a break from the constant updates.
  - Shut down those devices.
- **Avoid alcohol, caffeine and nicotine.**
  - Don't consume alcohol, or stimulating drinks like coffee or caffeinated teas or smoke right before you head to bed.
- **Seek help if you're struggling to cope.**
  - Talk to a mental health provider.
  - If you feel like you can't alleviate your stress and anxiety, or you have suicidal thought, call the National Suicide Prevention Lifeline 1-800-273-TALK (8255). https://suicidepreventionlifeline.org/

"The best way to find yourself is to lose yourself in the service of others."
- Mahatma Gandhi

- **Help Others to Help Your Heart!**
  - Scientific evidence shows that people who volunteer are 40% less likely to develop hypertension than non-volunteers.
- **Help Others to Lower Your Stress!**
  - A 2010 study showed that people who donate to charity have lower cortisol levels - that's the hormone that causes stress, anxiety, panic and higher blood pressure levels.
  - During this crisis, there are several ways you can help others. The Center for Disaster Philanthropy has set up the CDP COVID-19 Response Fund.
  - Check out the Charity Navigator for additional organizations and groups providing relief to others during the Coronavirus Pandemic.

EMOTIONAL WELLNESS

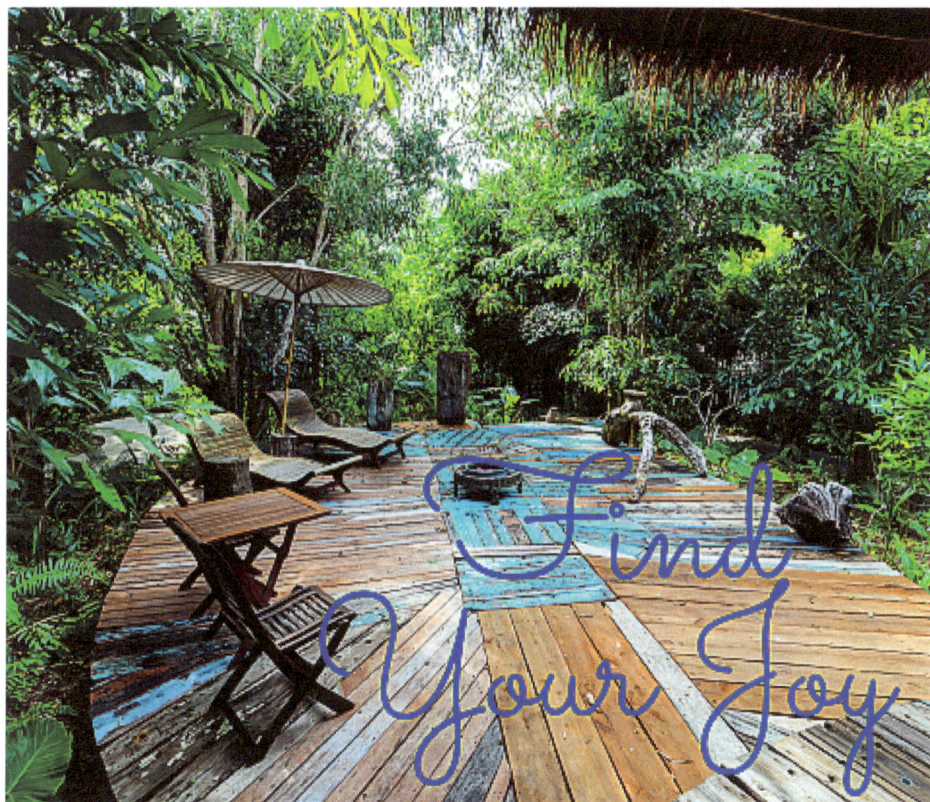

The COVID-19 Pandemic helped us to take a huge step forward and helped us uncover opportunities for improvement and understanding of what we need for future wellness. The journey to wellness starts with an intentional first step. Are you on the right path? Is your mind, body, and spirit in alignment?

Take this self-assessment to get your Wellness Quotient so you can define your focus to:
Get Well, Be Well, Stay Well.

EmWQ

EMOTIONAL WELLNESS - EmWQ

– Emotional Wellness means that you manage your emotions. You understand your feelings. You are aware of and respect the way others feel. And generally, you feel positive about your life.

1. I rarely have negative feelings, i.e. blue mood, despair, depression.
___1__ That's not me. I struggle with negative feelings, blue moods, despair, and depression.
___2__ Sometimes, but I manage it.
___3__ Often that's an issue for me.
___4__ That's me for sure! I am generally positive and upbeat.

2. I manage stress and can easily decompress without engaging in behaviors like binge eating or overeating, drinking, taking drugs, or engaging in other destructive actions.
__1___ That's not me. Stress is a big problem that I battle all the time.
__2___ Sometimes, I use food, alcohol, drugs, or other things to deal with my stress.
__3___ Often, stress drives me to do some unhealthy behaviors.
__4___ That's me a lot of times. I am good with dealing with stress and anxiety!

3. I know what I can control and what I cannot, and I can easily let go of things that are out of my control.
__1___ That's not me, I love to be in control and when I'm not, I get angry, upset, or worried.
__2___ Sometimes I get anxious about things I can't control.
__3___ Often, I am able to separate what's in my control and what's not.
__4___ That's me! I'm comfortable letting go of things beyond my control.

4. I cope with difficult feelings and confront them and work through them instead of avoiding them. __1___ That's not me, I run away from or avoid difficult feelings as much as possible.
__2___ Sometimes, I struggle with how to deal with difficult feelings.
__3___ Often, I am able to manage any difficult feelings.
__4___ Yes, I have ways to work through difficult feelings and I seek help if I need it.

5. I am aware of how other people feel.
__1___ That's not me. I have no idea how others feel.
__2___ Sometimes, I understand what others are feeling, but I could become more aware.
__3___ Often, I can relate to another person's feelings.
__4___ Yes, I regularly understand what others are feeling.

TOTAL FOR THIS SECTION ____

PHYSICAL WELLNESS

One of the eight tenets of overall wellness is Physical Wellness. In order to achieve physical wellness our bodies must be healthy and function well. We have to strike a balance between physical activity, proper nutrition, and mental well-being.

What is Physical Wellness?

Physical wellness is the care we give our bodies so we have optimal health and functioning.

Benefits of Physical Activity

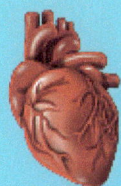

Healthy Heart

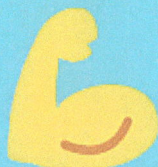

Improves Muscles/Joints

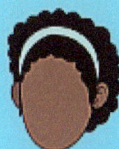

Firm & Supple Skin

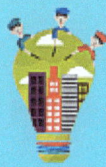

Improves Creativity

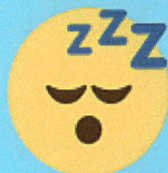

Improves Sleep

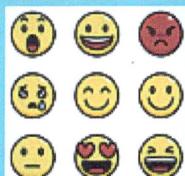

Improves Mood

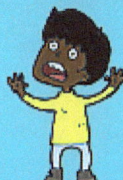

Reduces Stress

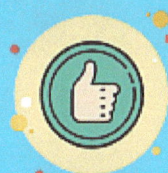

Increases Quality of Life

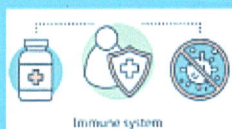

Boosts Immune System

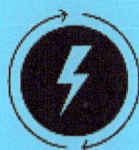

Increases Energy Levels

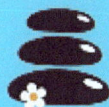

Improves Overall Wellbeing

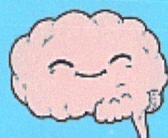

Stimulates Brain Plasticity

How Much Exercise Should I Do?

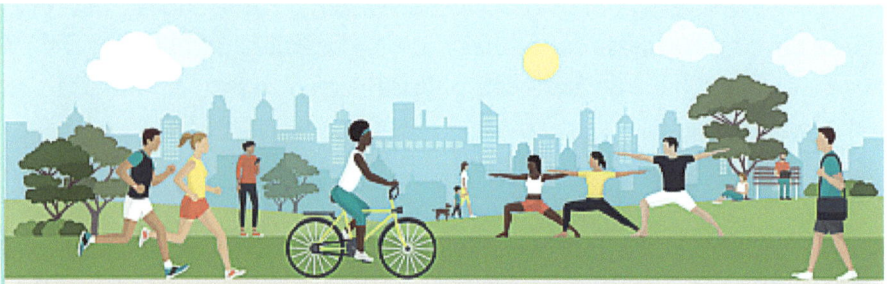

Get Well, Be Well, Stay Well - Let's Get Physical!

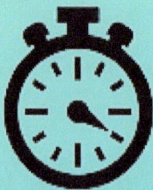

- **150** minutes of moderately intensive physical activity each week or **75** minutes of vigorously intensive activity each week (or equivalent combination).

- **300** minutes of moderately intensive physical activity for additional health benefits.

- **Anything that gets your heart beating faster** with rhythmic, large-muscle-group activity like walking, jogging, jumping rope, swimming, biking, aerobics, or dancing.

- Strength training of all major muscle groups - chest, back, shoulders, arms, lower back, abdominals, hips/thighs and calves at least **2-3 days** a week. (Resistance and/or weights)

- One to three sets (**eight to 15 repetitions per set**) each of **six to 10 exercises**.

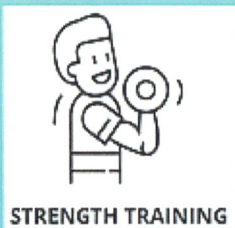

STRENGTH TRAINING

Additional Ways to Achieve Physical Wellness

- Eat a balanced diet

  - Eat 4 to 5 servings of fruits and vegetables daily.
  - Eat six servings of grains (at least half of them should be whole grains)
  - Have at least three servings of low fat or fat-free dairy daily.
  - Eat at least 8 to 9 servings per week of lean meat, poultry, and eggs.
  - Eat 2 to 3 servings of fish and seafood each week.
  - Eat 5 servings per week of nuts, seeds, beans, and legumes.

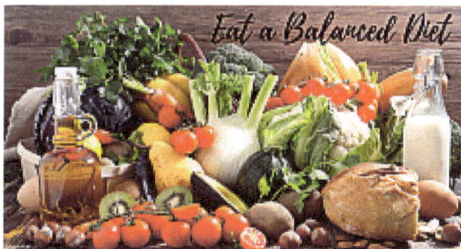

- Get regular sleep.

  - Most people need 7 to 9 hours per day to function well.

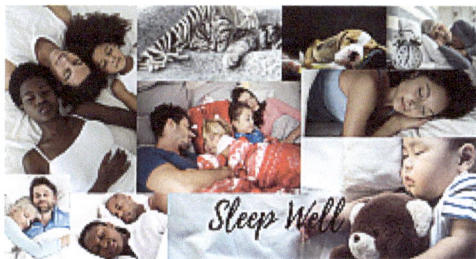

PWQ

PHYSICAL WELLNESS (PWQ)
– Physical Wellness is achieved through movement, physical activities, eating a balanced diet, and getting regular sleep.

1. I regularly do some sort of exercise two and a half hours per week or more when possible.
__1___ No, that's not me, I hate to exercise, or I don't make time to exercise.
__2___ Sometimes, I get some type of exercise in weekly.
__3___ Often, I incorporate exercise and physical activity into my weekly schedule.
__4___ Yes, I have a regular exercise routine and I faithfully stick to it!

2. I opt to walk or take the stairs when available.
__1___ That's not me at all – give me an elevator or escalator every time!
__2___ Sometimes, I opt to go for a walk and use stairs when I can.
__3___ Often, I regularly take walks and use stairs when possible.
__4___ Yes, that's me. I love to walk, and I park farther away to get my steps in!

3. I sit a lot for my job, so I give myself regular breaks every 30 minutes to get up, stretch, and move.
__1___ No, that's not me! If I am sitting, I am there for a long time.
__2___ Sometimes, I incorporate breaks to get up and move a bit.
__3___ Often, I get up, stand, stretch, and move.
__4___ Yes, I must keep active.

4. I wake up feeling rested and refreshed.
__1___ That's definitely not me! I feel sluggish when I wake up.
__2___ Sometimes, but not every day.
__3___ Often, I feel rested, refreshed, and ready for the day.
__4___ Oh, yes, that's me! I always wake up with a renewed sense of vigor.

5. I make an effort to eat a healthy, balanced diet that includes fruits an vegetables.
__1___ No, that's not me - I tend to eat a lot of junk food.
__2___ Sometimes, I eat healthy foods, but I could do better.
__3___ Often, I make healthy choices and eat moderate portions.
__4___ Yes, I maintain a strict diet that is well-balanced and healthy.

TOTAL FOR THIS SECTION _____

ENVIRONMENTAL WELLNESS

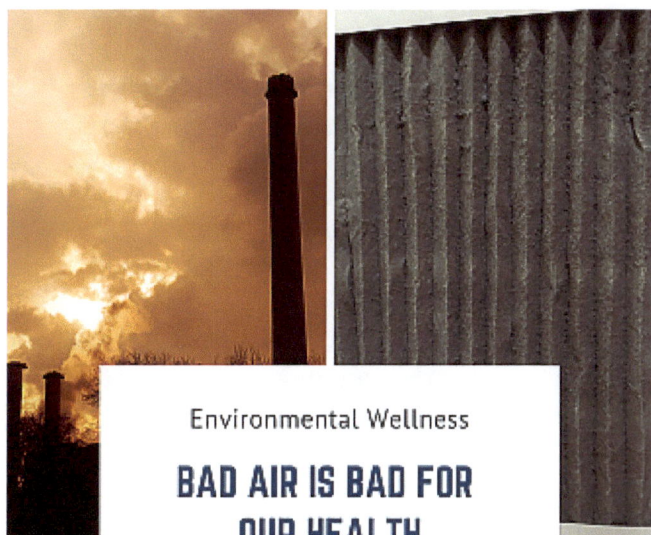

Environmental Wellness

BAD AIR IS BAD FOR OUR HEALTH

Overall Wellness

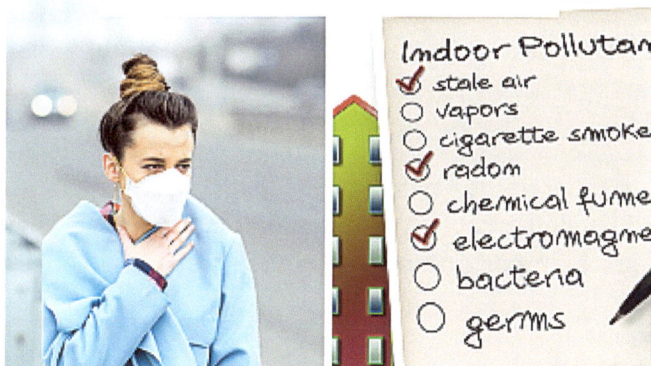

Indoor Pollutan
☑ stale air
○ vapors
○ cigarette smoke
☑ radon
○ chemical fume
☑ electromagne
○ bacteria
○ germs

What is Environmental Wellness?

Environmental wellness inspires us to live a lifestyle that is respectful of our surroundings. To enjoy environmental wellness we have to live harmoniously with the earth and do things to protect it. Environmental wellness also includes how well you interact with nature and your personal environment.

ENVIRONMENTAL WELLNESS

When the pandemic started, we heard that people with asthma and other compromised respiratory conditions were at higher risk of getting very ill from the virus. Now however, initial studies in the areas hardest hit by COVID-19 suggest that people who have experienced long-term exposure to pollution are at a greater risk of dying from Coronavirus.

Places right here in the U.S, like New York, Los Angeles, San Francisco, Chicago, Detroit as well as other countries known for pollution like China and Europe, have been hit especially hard.

These studies point to the fact that while this year we commemorated the 50th anniversary of Earth Day, we as global citizens, need to keep fighting for and demanding that we have clean air to breathe.

Yes, there have been some reports that during our social distancing some areas have actually seen their air quality improve. But what happens when the world starts gathering together again?

When this pandemic is over, don't forget that our attention to environmental wellness could save more lives in the future. And our indoor air quality is just as important to our overall health and well-being.

ENVIRONMENTAL WELLNESS

Biggest contributors to bad air inside our homes and businesses:

- Cigarette Smoke
- Particulates from candles and incense
- Perfumes
- Allergens, such as mold, pollen, pet dander, and dust mites.
- Art and office supplies, such as paints, glues, and toner ink.
- Wood-burning fireplaces or stoves.
- Building materials used in older homes like asbestos and lead.

Ways to Stay Healthy Indoors:

- Avoid smoking indoors (or quit all together!)
- Limit or avoid burning scented candles.
- Use arts and crafts in well-ventilated areas.
- Make sure gas stoves are vented properly.
- Remove carpeting, if possible.
- Use a dehumidifier and/or air conditioning to reduce moisture.
- Keep trash covered to avoid pests.
- Remove shoes at the door.
- Minimize the use of air fresheners.
- Use radon and carbon monoxide detectors.
- Fix leaky faucets
- Dust surfaces and vacuum frequently.
- Wash bedding weekly
- Make sure exhaust fans function properly.
- Exchange air inside with some fresh air from outside, if possible.

EnvWQ

ENVIRONMENTAL WELLNESS (EnvWQ)

– Environmental wellness means that you live a life that respects your surroundings. When you are environmentally well you live in harmony with the earth by doing things to protect it and understanding your impact with nature. It also means protecting your personal environment and taking action to protect the world around you.

1. I am aware of things I can do to improve my environmental impact on the earth.
__1___ No, that's not me, I really don't know how one person can make a difference to the earth.
__2___ Sometimes, I do things that will improve my impact on the earth, but I can do more.
__3___ Often I do things like opting to walk, ride a bike, or take public transportation instead of driving my own vehicle.
__4___ Yes, that's me! I know that every single person can do something to make a positive impact on the earth.

2. I use harmful chemicals sparingly around my home and properly dispose of them.
__1___ No, that's not me. I don't pay much attention to what chemicals are in the products I use.
__2___ Sometimes, I read labels and look for ways to get rid of products that could pose a problem.
__3___ Often I watch what chemicals I consume or use and find ways to correctly dispose of them.
__4___ Yes, that's me! I try to use natural products and things that are healthy for me, my family, my pets, and the earth.

3. I recycle and compost when I can and like to garden to improve my community.
__1___ No, that's not me. I am not sure why recycling, composting, and gardening make a difference.
__2___ Sometimes, I recycle things, when it's convenient to do so.
__3___ Often I have a refillable water bottle with me, so I don't have to get a bottle of water.
__4___ Yes, that's me! I reuse, recycle, and try to do things that are sustainable to the air and water resources.

4. I don't smoke, vape, or chew tobacco products so that I am healthy and that I protect others.
__1___ No, that's not me. Smoking, vaping, and chewing are my personal choices.
__2___ Sometimes, I try to stop smoking, but it's hard.
__3___ Often I go places where smoking, vaping, and chewing tobacco are not permitted.
__4___ Yes, that's me! I choose to engage in healthy activities for both me and the environment.

5. I keep my home and workplaces clean and clutter-free.
__1___ No, that's not me. I hate to clean, and I have junk everywhere.
__2___ Sometimes, I clean up, but I can definitely do better.
__3___ Often I clean my house and workspace, and I donate, or dispose of junk.
__4___ Yes, that's me! I want everything to be sparkling clean for my health and safety

TOTAL FOR THIS SECTION ____

OCCUPATIONAL WELLNESS

Being Well at Work Means More than Physical Wellness

As our communities, states, and the world begin to loosen restrictions from the COVID-19 Pandemic, many businesses will reopen and workers who were furloughed or laid-off may return to their previous jobs.

But for many jobless people, it may not be as simple as returning to the job they had prior to the pandemic. The world and rules will be different as a result of this complex health concern and the devastating economic impacts.

As business owners evaluate what the pandemic has done to their bottom line, they will also determine how best to move their companies forward and that could mean with fewer locations and a reduced workforce.

Safety on the job is on the minds of employers, as well as employees. Occupational wellness should be the focus for both.

So, what is Occupational Wellness?

Occupational wellness means having a career that is interesting, inspiring, and motivating. When workers use all of their talents, skills, and abilities, they perform better.

As the following checklist suggests, Occupational Wellness is much bigger than just physical well-being on the job.

OCCUPATIONAL WELLNESS

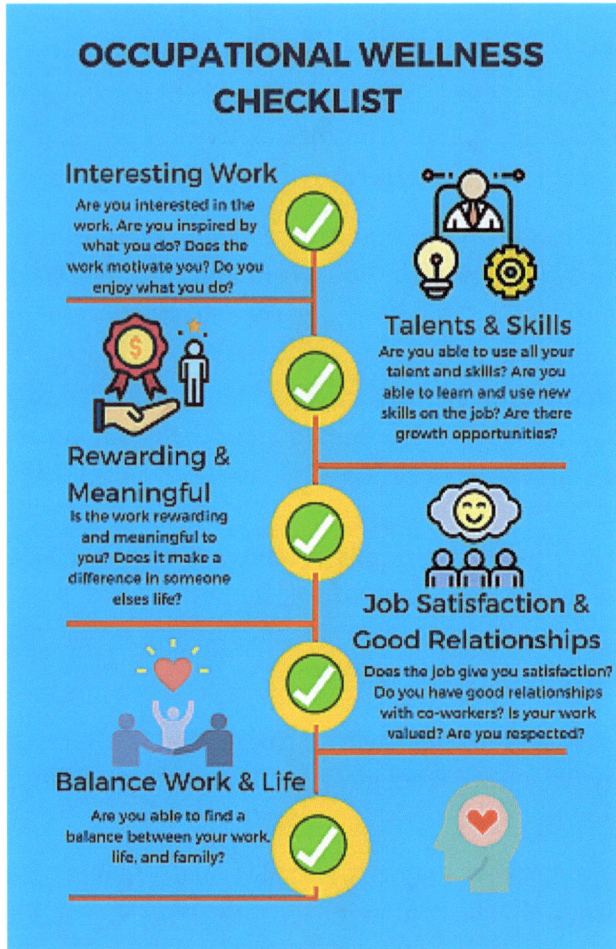

Ways to Promote Occupational Wellness in the Workplace

1. Employers should offer opportunities for employees to learn new skills.
2. Employees should seek growth opportunities.
3. Employers need to provide financially rewarding jobs and appreciate and recognize workers for their contributions.
4. Employers should offer a job or career that enables workers to balance work, family obligations, and personal interests.
5. Employees who are valued and respected enjoy greater job satisfaction.

www.bmiwellnessconcepts.com

OCCUPATIONAL WELLNESS

Now that mothers, fathers, grandparents, and children have been forced to work and learn under one roof due to the COVID-19 stay safe at home orders, employers got to see just how challenging it is to juggle life.

A post-pandemic workplace will require employers to be more sensitive, more accommodating, and even push employees toward finding balance if the employers want to have and retain a productive workforce.

Tips for Workers Seeking Occupational Wellness

- Don't settle.
    - Even if you've been out of work, don't settle for just anything.
    - You deserve a job that is interesting and inspirational.
- Keep motivated
    - Work toward what you want.
- Increase knowledge and skills.
    - Embrace any challenges directly.
- Enjoy what you do, do what you enjoy
    - Joy is something that you choose, regardless of the circumstances that you face.
- Find the benefits and positives in your current job.
    - Even if it's not your perfect job, find something positive about it.
    - Appreciate any benefit and anything positive, no matter if it is big or small.
- Create connections.
    - Connect with co-workers.
    - Network with others in your chosen field.
    - Seek out contacts in areas where you want to expand.
- Set goals.
    - Write down what you want to achieve.
    - Determine a plan to execute it.
    - Start implementing steps to achieve your goals.
- Seek career counseling.
    - If you want to try something new, look for someone to help you get there.
    - Don't be afraid to reach out and try something different.

OWQ

OCCUPATIONAL WELLNESS (OWQ)

– Occupational Wellness means that you are doing something that fully uses your talents and skills and it enriches your life. You find the work to be rewarding, fulfilling, satisfying, and meaningful. It aligns with your beliefs, values, and the goals you have set forth for your life.

1. I make a valuable and meaningful contribution to my community and the world through my work. __1___ No, that's not me. The work I do is just a job and a means to an end.
__2___ Sometimes, the work I do brings value and meaning to my community and the world.

__3___ Often I feel acknowledged for the work I do.
__4___ Yes, I know that the work I do is making a difference in the lives of others.

2. The work I do fits with my values and beliefs.
__1___ No, that's not me. I hate my job – it goes against everything I believe in, but it pays the bills. __2___ Sometimes, I feel that my values and beliefs align with the work I do.
__3___ Often, I am pleased to see just how well my values and beliefs fit with the work I do.
__4___ Yes, that's me – I am definitely in the right type of work for my values and beliefs.

3. My work is more than just a paycheck, it gives me great joy and a sense of accomplishment.

__1___ No, that's not me. My job is all about the money and I am ok with that.
__2___ Sometimes, the work I do is more than just money for me.
__3___ Often I receive joy and satisfaction knowing that what I do makes a difference to someone. __4___ Yes, that's me! I love the work I do, and I'd do it even if I wasn't getting paid.

4. I work in a field or area that allows me to showcase my talents and expertise.
__1___ No, that's not me, I know my talents, expertise would be valued somewhere else.
__2___ Sometimes, I feel that I get to showcase my talents and expertise, but I want more.
__3___ Often I get to do what I am really good at and what I really like to do.
__4___ Yes, that's me! I regularly get to showcase my talents and knowledge, and I am rewarded for it.

5. The work I do is important and therefore I always do my best.
__1___ No, that's not me – I do a thankless job and sometimes I slack off because no one cares.
__2___ Sometimes, the work I do is meaningful, so I try to do a good job.
__3___ Often I feel appreciated for the work I do, so I want to do as well as I can.
__4___ That's me for sure! I love my job, it gives me a sense of purpose and I seek to do my best!

TOTAL FOR THIS SECTION ____

FINANCIAL WELLNESS

Staying Financially Well During a Crisis is Critical to Your Overall Wellness

The dramatic and swift shift in our US and global economies due to the COVID-19 or Coronavirus Pandemic, has led to millions of people being furloughed, or losing their jobs. For many business owners, it means shutting down temporarily or closing for good.

If you live paycheck to paycheck, the financial strain is immediate. If you're fortunate enough to have a financial cushion, then you may be able to withstand the worst effects for a while.

But you have to find ways to stay financially well during this or any other crisis because your overall health and well-being depend on it!

What is Financial Wellness?

Financial wellness means that you are able to manage your economic life. That is that you are living within your means and paying all your expenses. It also means that you are financially prepared for emergencies. Having financial wellness means that you have access to information, tools, and resources to make financially sound decisions for the present and you have a plan for your future.

Financial wellness also provides people with the freedom to make choices about how and where you spend your money and it opens opportunities for what you want to do and where you want to go.

FINANCIAL WELLNESS

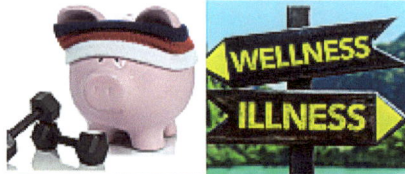

Get Financially Fit For Overall Wellness *(Even in a Crisis)*

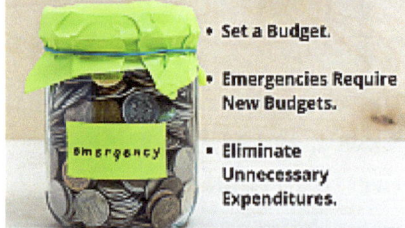

- Set a Budget.
- Emergencies Require New Budgets.
- Eliminate Unnecessary Expenditures.

Manage Financial Stress

Stress Increases:
- Blood Cholesterol
- Triglycerides
- Blood Sugar
- Blood Pressure
- Risks for Heart Disease

Diabetes, Depression, Sleep Disorders, Ulcers & Other Health Ailments

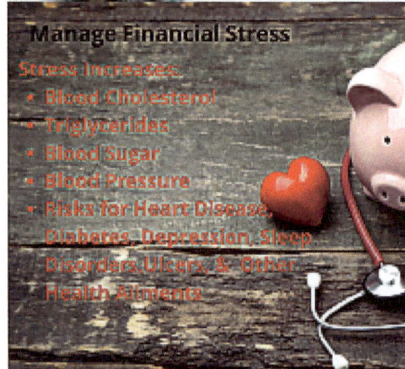

Be Mindful of Your Money
- Intentionally Pay Attention.
- Accept & Forgive Past Money Mistakes.
- Visualize and Plan for New Financial Success.
- Create and Empower More Supportive Spending Habits.

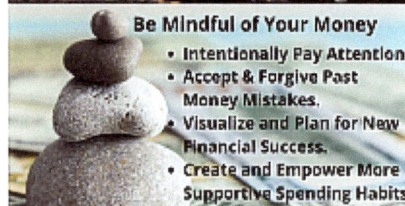

The CARES (Coronavirus Aid, Relief, and Economic Security) Act has many ways to help people and businesses during this pandemic with fast and direct relief. Take advantage of every relief option for which you may qualify. Many people received some Economic Impact Payments from the IRS. Before making any hasty decisions regarding your stocks, 401(k) and other retirement funds, please talk to your financial consultants on your best options.

www.bmiwellnessconcepts.com

FWQ

FINANCIAL WELLNESS (FWQ)

– Financial Wellness means that you are living a life of abundance. It doesn't mean that you are a millionaire, but that you are able to withstand a financial crisis, and that you have a plan for how you will pay your bills, so you aren't stressed over money. Financial wellness also provides a sense of security and the freedom to do things you want to do and to go places you want to go. Financial wellness also enables you to do things for others.

1. I am financially secure knowing that I can cover all my bills, and some of my wants.
__1___ No, that's not me! I am living paycheck-to-paycheck and some bills often go unpaid.
__2___ Sometimes I can indulge in something I want after all the bills are paid.
__3___ Often I am able to cover all my expenses and even indulge in a few splurges.
__4___ Yes, that's me, I am living comfortably financially.

2. I am living debt-free and able to live my best life.
__1___ No, that's not me! I have a lot of debt and don't know how to get out from under it.
__2___ Sometimes, I am able to manage my debts, but I could do better.
__3___ Often I am covering all my expenses and on track to be debt-free soon.
__4___ That's me – I have found a way to free myself and my family from the burden of debts.

3. I have a savings account and I regularly contribute to it.
__1___ No, that's not me! Savings account? I barely have any money in my checking account.
__2___ Sometimes, I am able to put a little money away in savings, but I want to do better.
__3___ Often I make regular deposits into a savings account.
__4___ Yes, that's me. I am a big saver. I want to know that my financial future is intact. If I were to lose my job tomorrow, I have enough saved to cover my expenses for five months.

4. I understand and manage my finances.
__1___ No, that's not me – If I need money, I go to the payday lender.
__2___ Sometimes, I manage my finances ok, but have on occasion borrowed money from friends and family.
__3___ Often I am looking for new ways to understand my finances and I have sought help from a financial planner.
__4___ Yes, this is me. I am on track for my retirement and I have dabbled in the stock market.

5. I live within my means and only purchase things I can truly afford.
__1___ No, that's not me, If I have money, it burns a hole in my pocket. And my charge card is my friend.
__2___ Sometimes, but I occasionally reward myself with a guilty pleasure.
__3___ Often I try not to pay with a credit card and only pay for things with the money that's directly in my account.
__4___ Yes, this is me, I understand the value of money and always try to get the most bang for my buck and I don't try to live like the Jones'.

TOTAL FOR THIS SECTION ___

WQ

TOTAL WELLNESS QUOTIENT

It is important to your overall well-being that you work to maintain these eight tenets of wellness into your daily life.

Intellectual Wellness
To achieve intellectual wellness open your mind to new experiences and new ideas. Expand your knowledge. Refine your skills. Participate in activities that stimulate your thoughts. Enhance your understanding of different cultures. Embrace your artistic expression. Foster your creativity. Be curious. Develop mindfulness, and learn something new every day.

Social Wellness
To achieve social wellness pay attention to how well you relate and connect with others. Even if you have to maintain some physical distance in a pandemic, you still need to have some meaningful interactions with your family and friends. But you also need to make sure that your community experiences social wellness, too. That means that everyone is valued and treated with respect.

Spiritual Wellness
To achieve spiritual wellness, connect to something greater than yourself. Develop a spiritual set of values, principles, morals and beliefs that give you a sense of purpose and meaning and help guide your life. Meditate, pray, and find what grounds you.

Emotional Wellness
As you work to achieve emotional wellness, you will develop coping mechanisms to effectively deal with life's challenges. With emotional wellness, you have to build healthy relationships with others, so you feel confident and in control of your feelings and behaviors.

WELLNESS QUOTIENT - WQ

Physical Wellness

To achieve physical wellness, you must care for your body, so you have optimal health and it functions well for you. Eat a balanced diet. Exercise daily, even if it is something as simple as taking a walk, going on a run or a bike ride. Also, make sure to get enough sleep to replenish your mind and body.

Environmental Wellness

To enjoy environmental wellness we have to live harmoniously with the earth and do things to protect it. Environmental wellness also involves how well you interact with nature and your personal environment. So, just as the air and water outside must be maintained for the natural environments, pay attention to the air you breathe inside, too. Make sure it is healthy for you, your family, and your pets.

Occupational Wellness

To achieve occupational wellness, you have to find a career that is interesting, inspiring, and motivating. When you are able to use all of your talents, skills, and abilities, you will undoubtedly perform better on the job!

Financial Wellness

To achieve financial wellness, you have to manage your economic life. You live within your means and pay all of your expenses. You are financially prepared for emergencies. Experiencing financial wellness means that you have access to information, tools, and resources to make financially sound decisions for the present and you have a plan for your future.

Now, go back and get the totals for each wellness section and add them here to find out your Wellness Quotient (WQ)

WELLNESS QUOTIENT - WQ

WELLNESS QUOTIENT	SURVEY SCORE
INTELLECTUAL WELLNESS (IWQ)	____
SOCIAL WELLNESS (SoWQ)	____
SPIRITUAL WELLNESS (SpWQ)	____
EMOTIONAL WELLNESS (EmWQ)	____
PHYSICAL WELLNESS (PWQ)	____
ENVIRONMENTAL WELLNESS (EnvWQ)	____
OCCUPATIONAL WELLNESS (OWQ)	____
FINANCIAL WELLNESS (FWQ)	____
TOTAL WELLNESS (TWQ)	____

WHAT YOUR WELLNESS QUOTIENT MEANS:

40 – 80 There are a lot of ways for you to improve your overall wellness by being intentional, focused, and by seeking balance in your life.

81 - 100 You have an idea about how to achieve wellness, you just need to make it a priority in your life.

101 - 125 You are already working hard on your wellness initiatives, with a few more intentional efforts, you will be able to find a healthy balance in your life.

126 -160 You are living a life of wellness, balance, and harmony. What else would you like to achieve? Or how can you help others increase their overall wellness?

To improve your Wellness Quotient, let us be your first destination on your wellness journey to

GET WELL, BE WELL, STAY WELL.

SUMMARY

Summary

A pandemic usually means an outbreak of a disease such as COVID-19, that occurs over a wide geographic area - like the world. A "disease" must also be infectious in order to be a pandemic.

Sadly, both COVID-19 and social injustice qualify as pandemics. Like the Black Lives Matter movement created in the US, BMI Wellness Concepts wants to "be the change" (Mahatma Ghandi) to help you identify your Wellness Quotient (WQ)and to ultimately create a Wellness Pandemic within you and throughout the world.

Dr. Sherri James, MD and BMI Wellness Concepts provide people with affordable pathways to achieving overall wellness for long, happy, healthy lives. BMI Wellness Concepts and FINDING WELLNESS IN A PANDEMIC AND BEYOND provided you with the tools to integrate your body and mind into alignment to **Get Well, Be Well, Stay Well!**

Enhance your wellness journey by taking the Wellness Quotient Survey and connecting with BMI Wellness Concepts.

WELLNESS SURVEY -IWQ

COMPLETE WELLNESS QUOTIENT SURVEY

iNSTRUCTIONS: Answer each question accurately. Each answer that describes you best, will be scored on a scale of 1 to 4: 1 = Nope, that is not me. 2 = Sometimes, that describes me. 3 = Often that is me. 4 = Yes, that's definitely me!

INTELLECTUAL WELLNESS - IWQ

- Intellectual Wellness has to do with how curious you are and how open you are to learn or experience new things. It includes embracing or tackling new challenges and finding ways to develop additional skills. It also has to do with your ability to share your knowledge and expertise with other.

1. I am curious about new topics, different cultures, and visiting places outside my community, region, or country.

__1___ No, that's not me, I am comfortable with what I know and where I live.
__2___ Sometimes, I am open to learning new things, meeting new people, and seeing new places.
__3___ Often I seek to learn about people, places, and cultures that are different from my life.
__4___ Yes! I want to experience as much as I can from many different people, cultures, and sources.

2. I regularly seek out activities that challenge my brain, stimulate my curiosity, or offer inspiration.

__1___ No, that's not me. I'm not one to really seek new experiences.
__2___ Sometimes I look for ways to make me think about things or see things from a different perspective.
__3___ Often I am curious, and I look for new ways of thinking about situations.
__4___ Yes, I constantly seek new challenges and my brain thrives on curiosity and inspiration!

3. I enjoy sharing my knowledge and expertise with others as a way of helping people.

__1___ No, that's not me. I don't feel like I have any knowledge or expertise that is valuable to others.
__2___ Sometimes, I like to share what I know or what I have experienced with others.
__3___ Often I look for ways that I can help people with my knowledge, expertise, and experiences.
__4___ Yes, I find satisfaction that my knowledge and expertise can help others.

4. When I learn new information, I am open to changing my mind or seeing a different perspective.

__1___ No, that's not me. I am comfortable knowing that I know what I need to know.
__2___ Sometimes, I am open to learning new information and considering a new way of thinking.
__3___ Often I seek out new ways of thinking about situations
__4___ Yes! I want to learn new information, hear different perspectives, and challenge my beliefs for my own growth.

5. When I make a mistake, I own it and I use it as a way to learn from it.

__1___ No, that's not me – I am sure that something or someone caused me to flub up.
__2___ Sometimes, I accept the errors I make and I'm willing to try to find a lesson in that mistake.
__3___ Often I accept my failings, and I make changes to prevent similar mistakes in the future.
__4___ Yes, I know when I mess up and I want to make sure that I don't do it again.

TOTAL FOR THIS SECTION ____

WELLNESS SURVEY - SoWQ

SOCIAL WELLNESS - SoWQ

– Social Wellness means that you cultivate and maintain connections and relationships with family, friends, and colleagues and that you are able to work through any conflicts that might arise.

1. I choose to spend time with people who know me best and with whom I am my best self.
__1___ No, that's not me, I always manage to find people in my life who don't respect me or hurt me.
__2___ Sometimes, I seek out healthy relationships with family, friends, and co-workers.
__3___ Often my family, friends, and co-workers build me up.
__4___ Yes, my family, friends, and co-workers and I are a great team.

2. I am comfortable with and appreciate my relationships within my community.
__1___ No, that's not me. My relationships are strained.
__2___ Sometimes, I feel comfortable with my relationships with family, friends, or co-workers.
__3___ Often, I seek comfort from my friends, family, and/or co-workers.
__4___ Yes, I need my friends and family and I love being a part of my community.

3. I'm comfortable in my skin and confident in my decisions.
__1___ No, that's not me – I'm a people-pleaser. I worry about what others think of me.
__2___ Sometimes, I am ruled by the need to please others.
__3___ Often, I can separate my need to always please others.
__4___ Yes, I'm a renegade. I know that I can't please everyone, and I am OK with that.

4. I am comfortable being alone.
__1___ No, that's not me. I can't stand being alone – I am very much a people person.
__2___ Sometimes, I isolate myself from friends, family, and co-workers.
__3___ Often I seek regular meetings and get-togethers with family and friends.
__4___ Yes, I may be alone, but I am not lonely.

5. I work hard to not lash out and blame others for my frustrations and anger.
__1___ No, I often blame others when I am frustrated or angry.
__2___ Sometimes, when I get frustrated or angry, I lash out at others.
__3___ Often I am able to keep frustrations and anger in check.
__4___ Yes, I take responsibility for my own actions, and I do not blame others for my frustrations and anger.

TOTAL FOR THIS SECTION ___

WELLNESS SURVEY - SpWQ

SPIRITUAL WELLNESS -SpWQ

– Spiritual wellness has to do with how meaningful your life is and whether you live a life that has purpose and is bolstered by your beliefs, faith, and morals.

1. I make choices in my life that are rewarding and fulfilling to me.
__1___ No, that's not me. I need to make better choices in my life.
__2___ Sometimes, I do things that give me a sense of accomplishment, but I could do more.
__3___ Often, I seek out ways to feel like I am making a difference in someone else's life.
__4___ Yes! I thrive on doing things that feed my soul and make me feel fulfilled.

2. I like being a part of something bigger than myself.
__1___ No, I prefer to be by myself and focus only on my own personal issues.
__2___ Sometimes, I seek out ways to be part of the larger community.
__3___ Often, I look for ways to get involved with new groups or things that are important to the community as a whole.
__4___ Yes, I thrive on being a part of meaningful activities that have a positive purpose.

3. I know what issues matters to me, and I keep them at the center of my life.
__1___ No, I struggle with finding a purpose or meaning to my life.
__2___ Sometimes I think I know what is important to me and I manage to stay on track with it.
__3___ Often I am centered and focused on what's important in my life.
__4___ Yes, I have discovered my passion and I never waiver in my pursuit.

4. I wake up with a sense of purpose and direction every day.
__1___ No, that's not me at all! My life has no meaning or purpose.
__2___ Sometimes I know what I am supposed to be doing and mostly I stay on track for that goal.
__3___ Often I am guided by what my purpose is in life.
__4___ Yes! I am on track and motivated to accomplish what I set out to do.

5. Everything I do coincides with my values, beliefs, faith, and life tenets.
__1___ No, that's not me – I really don't know what I value or what I believe.
__2___ Sometimes, I struggle to do things that fit within my beliefs or faith.
__3___ Often I set out to do things that align with what I value or hold dear to me.
__4___ Yes, I know what I believe and my faith in those beliefs guide and shape my life daily.

TOTAL FOR THIS SECTION ___

WELLNESS SURVEY - EmWQ

EMOTIONAL WELLNESS - EmWQ
– Emotional Wellness means that you manage your emotions. You understand your feelings. You are aware of and respect the way others feel. And generally, you feel positive about your life.

1. I rarely have negative feelings, i.e. blue mood, despair, depression?
___1__ That's not me. I struggle with negative feelings, blue moods, despair, and depression.
___2__ Sometimes, but I manage it.
___3__ Often that's an issue for me.
___4__ That's me for sure! I am generally positive and upbeat.

2. I manage stress and can easily decompress without engaging in behaviors like binge eating or overeating, drinking, taking drugs, or engaging in other destructive actions. _
__1___ That's not me. Stress is a big problem that I battle all the time.
__2___Sometimes, I use food, alcohol, drugs, or other things to deal with my stress.
__3___Often, stress drives me to do some unhealthy behaviors.
__4___ That's me a lot of times. I am good with dealing with stress and anxiety!

3. I know what I can control and what I cannot, and I can easily let go of things that are out of my control.
__1___ That's not me, I love to be in control and when I'm not, I get angry, upset, or worried
__2___ Sometimes I get anxious about things I can't control.
__3___ Often, I am able to separate what's in my control and what's not.
__4___ That's me! I'm comfortable letting go of things beyond my control.

4. I cope with difficult feelings and confront them and work through them instead of avoiding them.
__1___ That's not me, I run away from or avoid difficult feelings as much as possible.
__2___ Sometimes, I struggle with how to deal with difficult feelings.
__3___ Often, I am able to manage any difficult feelings.
__4___ Yes, I have ways to work through difficult feelings and I seek help if I need it.

5. I am aware of how other people feel.
__1___ That's not me. I have no idea how others feel.
__2___ Sometimes, I understand what others are feeling, but I could become more aware.
__3___ Often, I can relate to another person's feelings.
__4___ Yes, I regularly understand what others are feeling.

TOTAL FOR THIS SECTION ____

WELLNESS SURVEY - PWQ

PHYSICAL WELLNESS - PWQ

– Physical Wellness is achieved through movement, physical activities, eating a balanced diet, and getting regular sleep.

1. I regularly do some sort of exercise two and a half hours per week or more when possible.
__1___ No, that's not me, I hate to exercise, or I don't make time to exercise.
__2___ Sometimes, I get some type of exercise in weekly.
__3___ Often, I incorporate exercise and physical activity into my weekly schedule.
__4___ Yes, I have a regular exercise routine and I faithfully stick to it!

2. I opt to walk or take the stairs when available.
__1___ That's not me at all – give me an elevator or escalator every time!
__2___ Sometimes, I opt to go for a walk and use stairs when I can.
__3___ Often, I regularly take walks and use stairs when possible.
__4___ Yes, that's me. I love to walk, and I park farther away to get my steps in!

3. I sit a lot for my job, so I give myself regular breaks every 30 minutes to get up, stretch, and move.
__1___ No, that's not me! If I am sitting, I am there for a long time.
__2___ Sometimes, I incorporate breaks to get up and move a bit.
__3___ Often, I get up, stand, stretch, and move.
__4___ Yes, I must keep active.

4. I wake up feeling rested and refreshed.
__1___ That's definitely not me! I feel sluggish when I wake up.
__2___ Sometimes, but not every day.
__3___ Often, I feel rested, refreshed, and ready for the day.
__4___ Oh, yes, that's me! I always wake up with a renewed sense of vigor.

5. I make an effort to eat a healthy, balanced diet that includes fruits and vegetables.
__1___ No, that's not me – I tend to eat a lot of junk food.
__2___ Sometimes, I eat healthy foods, but I could do better.
__3___ Often I make healthy choices and eat moderate portions.
__4___ Yes, I maintain a strict diet that is well-balanced and healthy.

TOTAL FOR THIS SECTION ____

WELLNESS QUOTIENT - EnvWQ

ENVIRONMENTAL WELLNESS - EnvWQ

– Environmental wellness means that you live a life that respects your surroundings. When you are environmentally well you live in harmony with the earth by doing things to protect it and understanding your impact with nature. It also means protecting your personal environment and taking action to protect the world around you.

1. I am aware of things I can do to improve my environmental impact on the earth.
__1___ No, that's not me, I really don't know how one person can make a difference to the earth.
__2___ Sometimes, I do things that will improve my impact on the earth, but I can do more.
__3___ Often I do things like opting to walk, ride a bike, or take public transportation instead of driving my own vehicle.
__4___ Yes, that's me! I know that every single person can do something to make a positive impact on the earth.

2. I use harmful chemicals sparingly around my home and properly dispose of them.
__1___ No, that's not me. I don't pay much attention to what chemicals are in the products I use.
__2___ Sometimes, I read labels and look for ways to get rid of products that could pose a problem.
__3___ Often I watch what chemicals I consume or use and find ways to correctly dispose of them.
__4___ Yes, that's me! I try to use natural products and things that are healthy for me, my family, my pets, and the earth.

3. I recycle and compost when I can and like to garden to improve my community.
__1___ No, that's not me. I am not sure why recycling, composting, and gardening make a difference.
__2___ Sometimes, I recycle things, when it's convenient to do so.
__3___ Often I have a refillable water bottle with me, so I don't have to get a bottle of water.
_4__ Yes, that's me! I reuse, recycle, and try to do things that are sustainable to the air and water resources.

4. I don't smoke, vape, or chew tobacco products so that I am healthy and that I protect others.
__1___ No, that's not me. Smoking, vaping, and chewing are my personal choices.
__2___ Sometimes, I try to stop smoking, but it's hard.
__3___ Often I go places where smoking, vaping, and chewing tobacco are not permitted.
__4___ Yes, that's me! I choose to engage in healthy activities for both me and the environment.

5. I keep my home and workplaces clean and clutter-free.
__1___ No, that's not me. I hate to clean, and I have junk everywhere.
_2___ Sometimes, I clean up, but I can definitely do better.
__3___ Often I clean my house and workspace, and I donate, or dispose of junk.
__4___ Yes, that's me! I want everything to be sparkling clean for my health and safety

TOTAL FOR THIS SECTION ____

WELLNESS QUOTIENT - OWQ

OCCUPATIONAL WELLNESS - OWQ
– Occupational Wellness means that you are doing something that fully uses your talents and skills and it enriches your life. You find the work to be rewarding, fulfilling, satisfying, and meaningful. It aligns with your beliefs, values, and the goals you have set forth for your life.

1. I make a valuable and meaningful contribution to my community and the world through my work.
_1___ No, that's not me. The work I do is just a job and a means to an end.
_2___ Sometimes, the work I do brings value and meaning to my community and the world.
_3___ Often I feel acknowledged for the work I do.
_4___ Yes, I know that the work I do is making a difference in the lives of others.

2. The work I do fits with my values and beliefs.
_1___ No, that's not me. I hate my job – it goes against everything I believe in, but it pays the bills.
_2___ Sometimes, I feel that my values and beliefs align with the work I do.
_3___ Often, I am pleased to see just how well my values and beliefs fit with the work I do.
_4___ Yes, that's me – I am definitely in the right type of work for my values and beliefs.

3. My work is more than just a paycheck, it gives me great joy and a sense of accomplishment.
_1___ No, that's not me. My job is all about the money and I am ok with that.
_2___ Sometimes, the work I do is more than just money for me.
_3___ Often I receive joy and satisfaction knowing that what I do makes a difference to someone.
_4___ Yes, that's me! I love the work I do, and I'd do it even if I wasn't getting paid.

4. I work in a field or area that allows me to showcase my talents and expertise.
_1___ No, that's not me, I know my talents, expertise would be valued somewhere else.
_2___ Sometimes, I feel that I get to showcase my talents and expertise, but I want more.
_3___ Often I get to do what I am really good at and what I really like to do.
_4___ Yes, that's me! I regularly get to showcase my talents and knowledge, and I'm rewarded for it.

5. The work I do is important and therefore I always do my best.
_1___ No, that's not me – I do a thankless job and sometimes I slack off because no one cares.
_2___ Sometimes, the work I do is meaningful, so I try to do a good job.
_3___ Often I feel appreciated for the work I do, so I want to do as well as I can.
_4___ That's me for sure! I love my job, it gives me a sense of purpose and I seek to do my best!

TOTAL FOR THIS SECTION ____

WELLNESS QUOTIENT - FWQ

FINANCIAL WELLNESS - FWQ

– Financial Wellness means that you are living a life of abundance. It doesn't mean that you are a millionaire, but that you are able to withstand a financial crisis, and that you have a plan for how you will pay your bills, so you aren't stressed over money. Financial wellness also provides a sense of security and the freedom to do things you want to do and to go places you want to go. Financial wellness also enables you to do things for others.

1. I am financially secure knowing that I can cover all my bills, and some of my wants.
__1___ No, that's not me! I am living paycheck-to-paycheck and some bills often go unpaid.
__2___ Sometimes I can indulge in something I want after all the bills are paid.
__3___ Often I am able to cover all my expenses and even indulge in a few splurges.
__4___ Yes, that's me, I am living comfortably financially.

2. I am living debt-free and able to live my best life.
__1___ No, that's not me! I have a lot of debt and don't know how to get out from under it.
__2___ Sometimes, I am able to manage my debts, but I could do better.
__3___ Often I am covering all my expenses and on track to be debt-free soon.
__4___ That's me – I have found a way to free myself and my family from the burden of debts.

3. I have a savings account and I regularly contribute to it.
__1___ No, that's not me! Savings account? I barely have any money in my checking account.
__2___ Sometimes, I am able to put a little money away in savings, but I want to do better.
__3___ Often I make regular deposits into a savings account.
__4___ Yes, that's me. I am a big saver. I want to know that my financial future is intact. If I were to lose my job tomorrow, I have enough saved to cover my expenses for five months.

4. I understand and manage my finances.
__1___ No, that's not me – If I need money, I go to the payday lender.
__2___ Sometimes, I manage my finances ok, but have on occasion borrowed money from friends and family.
__3___ Often I am looking for new ways to understand my finances and I have sought help from a financial planner.
__4___ Yes, this is me. I am on track for my retirement and I have dabbled in the stock market.

5. I live withing my means and only purchase things that I can truly afford.
__1___ No, that's not me, If I have money, it burns a hole in my pocket. And my charge card is my friend.
__2___ Sometimes, but I occasionally reward myself with a guilty pleasure.
__3___ Often I try not to pay with a credit card and only pay for things with the money that's directly in my account.
__4___ Yes, this is me, I understand the value of money and always try to get the most bang for my buck and I don't try to live like the Jones'.

TOTAL FOR THIS SECTION ____

WELLNESS QUOTIENT - WQ

Now, go back and get the totals for each wellness section and add them here to find out your Wellness Quotient (WQ)

WELLNESS QUOTIENT	SURVEY SCORE
INTELLECTUAL WELLNESS (IWQ)	____
SOCIAL WELLNESS (SoWQ)	____
SPIRITUAL WELLNESS (SpWQ)	____
EMOTIONAL WELLNESS (EmWQ)	____
PHYSICAL WELLNESS (PWQ)	____
ENVIRONMENTAL WELLNESS (EnvWQ)	____
OCCUPATIONAL WELLNESS (OWQ)	____
FINANCIAL WELLNESS (OWQ)	____

WHAT YOUR WELLNESS QUOTIENT MEANS:

40 – 80 There are a lot of ways for you to improve your overall wellness by being intentional, focused, and by seeking balance in your life.

81 - 100 You have an idea about how to achieve wellness, you just need to make it a priority in your life.

101 - 125 You are already working hard on your wellness initiatives, with a few more intentional efforts, you will be able to find a healthy balance in your life.

126 -160 You are living a life of wellness, balance, and harmony. What else would you like to achieve? Or how can you help others increase their overall wellness?

To improve your Wellness Quotient, let us be your first destination on your wellness journey to

GET WELL, BE WELL, STAY WELL.

For the online Wellness Quotient Survey visit www.bmiwellnessconcepts.com

BMI WELLNESS CONCEPTS, PLLC

ABOUT BMI WELLNESS CONCEPTS

Sherri James, MD and BMI Wellness Concepts are committed to facilitating transformation to eradicate chronic disease so people can achieve optimal health and wellness.

Fewer Prescription Drugs With Greater Body, Mind Alignment

BMI Wellness Concepts...

An affordable destination on your wellness journey!

Conditions and Illnesses We Treat:

Chronic fatigue and low energy

Brain fog

Blood sugar problems/diabetes

Digestive problems

Diets and detox

Immune disorders

Depression / anxiety

Joint pain / arthritis

Obesity

Headaches

Blood pressure

Cholesterol / Heart disease

Fibromyalgia

Menopause - female and male

Hormone imbalance - male and female

CONNECT WITH BMI WELLNESS CONCEPTS

Phone:	844-4WELLNS
	844-493-5567
Tele-Wellness:	844-TELWELL
	844-835-9355
Wellness Parties	844-4PRTWLL
	844-477-8955
Email:	info@bmiwellnessconcepts.com

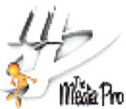

Contributing Author and Creative Design:
Jill Hammergren, The Media Pro
https://themediapro.biz/
jill@themediapro.biz

www.bmiwellnessconcepts.com

MEET THE AUTHOR

ABOUT THE AUTHOR, SHERRI JAMES, MD

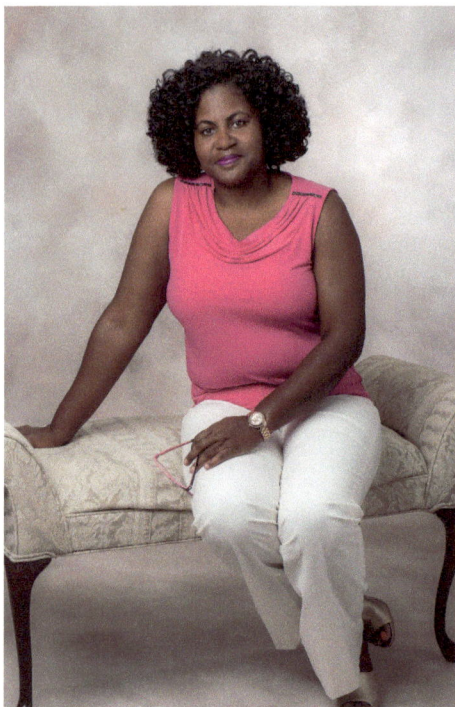

Sherri James, MD
Owner, BMI Wellness Concepts, LLC

Dr. Sherri James is currently the Founder and Owner of an integrative medicine practice known as BMI Wellness Concepts, PLLC. She has more than 25 years of diverse leadership and practical experience as a family doctor. Her career spans across several medical sectors including Federally Qualified Community Health Centers, public health, rural medicine, occupational medicine and opioid dependency. She initially earned a BS in Pharmacy from the Florida A&M University and later earned an MD degree from the University of Miami.

She went on to complete a Family Medicine Residency at UT Houston, a Rural Medicine Fellowship in Shreveport, LA and East Texas, a Masters in Healthcare Administration from UT Dallas and certification as a Professional Health Coach from the Duke Integrative Medicine Institute. As a physician and wellness advocate, she strives to educate patients according to a "wellness model" rather than the traditional "sick model" of healthcare as we know it today in the United States. By so doing, she hopes to eliminate health disparities and to make our communities both healthy and wealthy - because your health is your greatest wealth. Her motto is:

GET WELL, BE WELL, STAY WELL

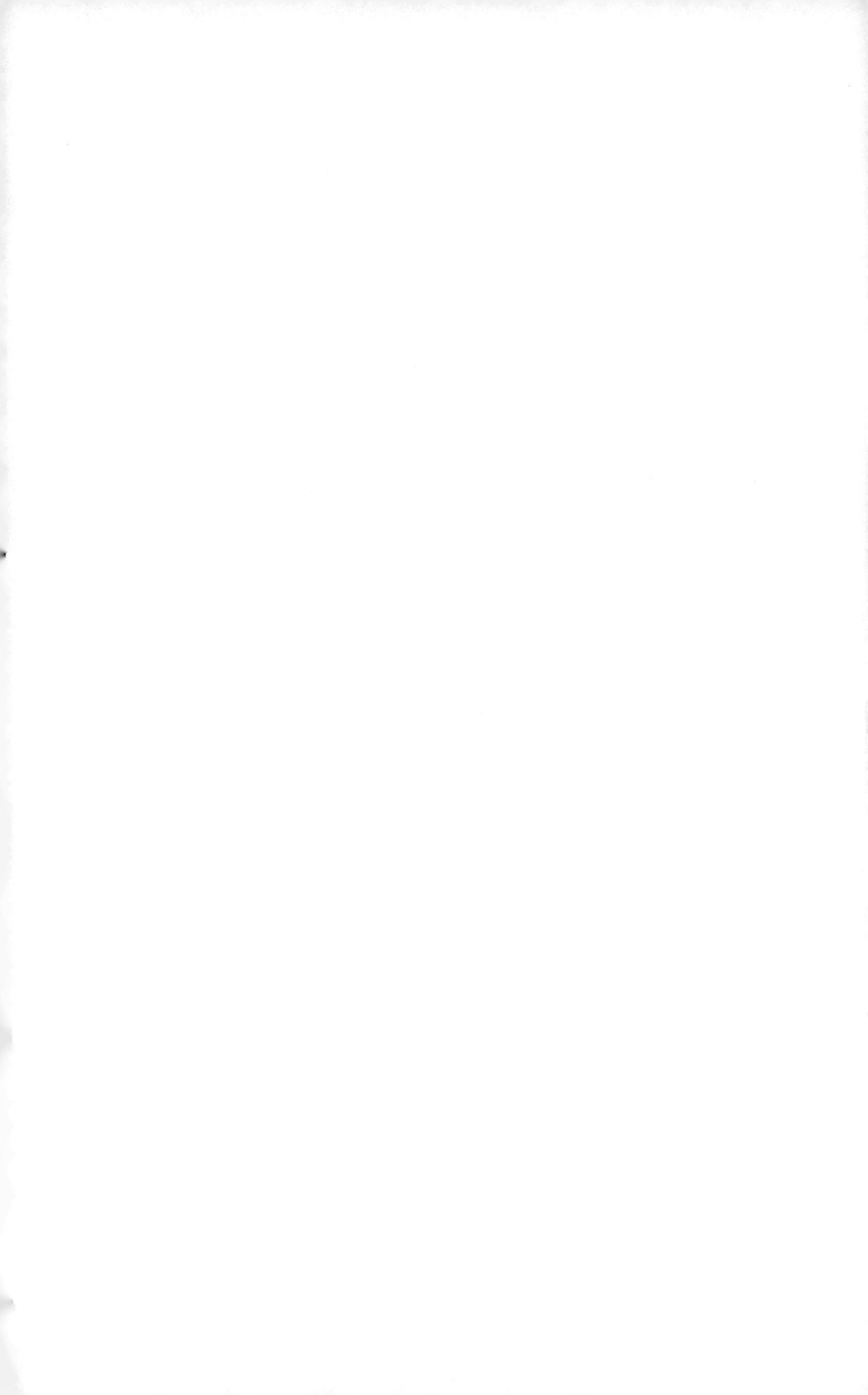

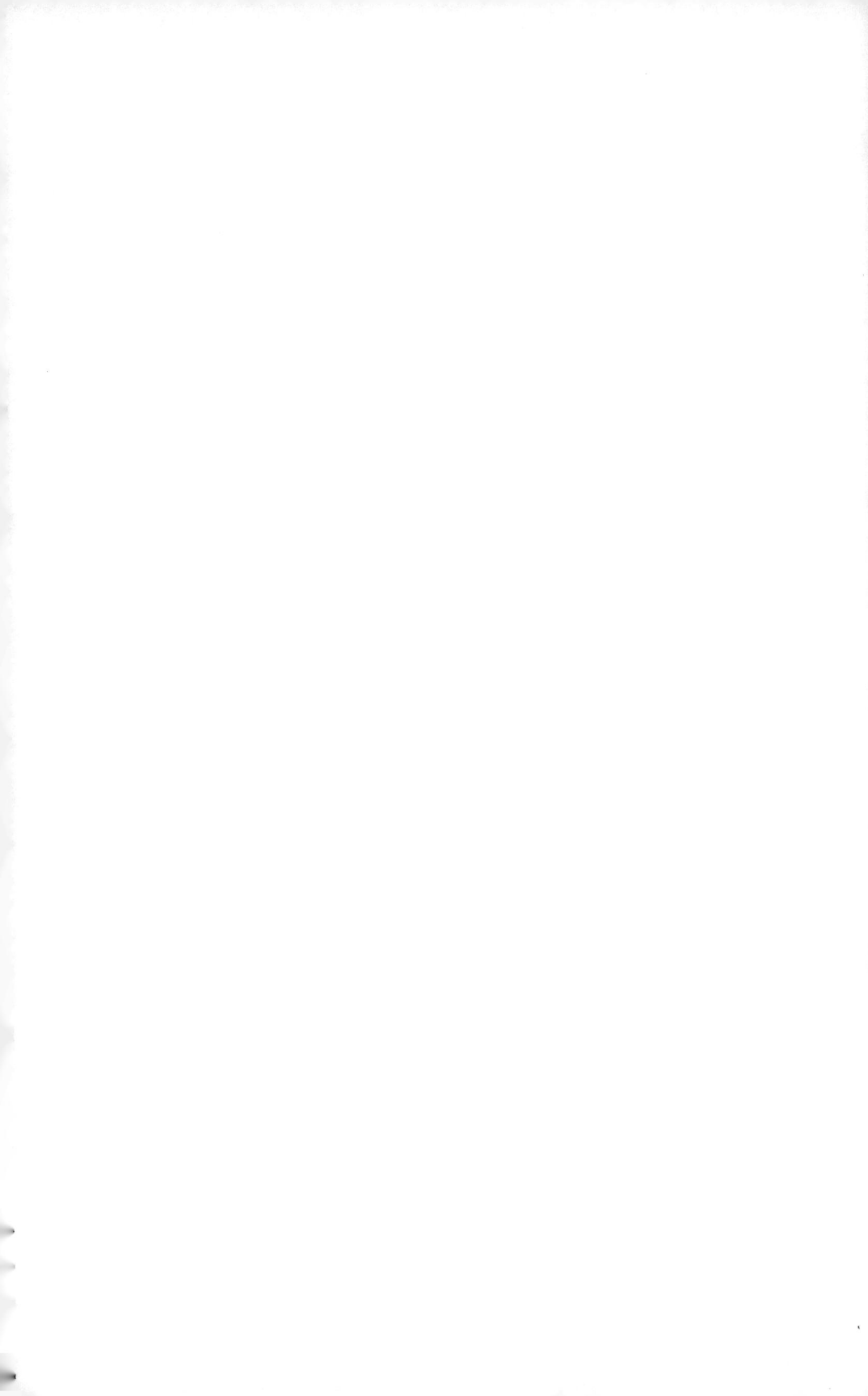

www.ingramcontent.com/pod-product-compliance
Lightning Source LLC
Chambersburg PA
CBHW040932030426
42336CB00001B/8